« A Family Guide to Wellness »

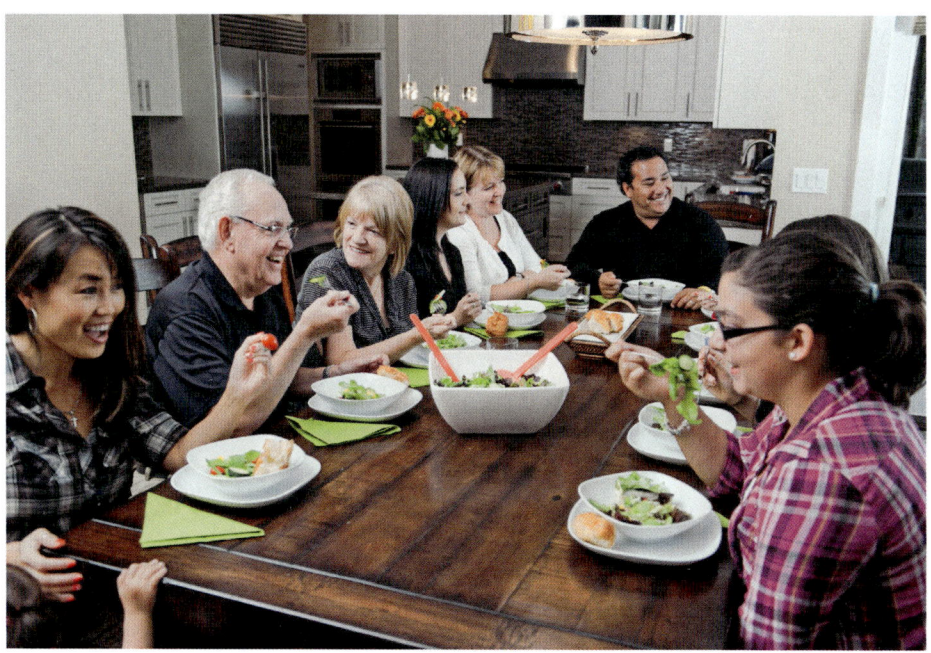

Judd Allen, Ph.D.

President, Human Resources Institute, LLC

« Contents »

The Family and Wellness Connection..5

Topic 1: Getting Comfortable with Family Wellness...................7

Topic 2: Seeing Your Unique Family System..............................8

Topic 3: Developing Your Family's Wellness Story.....................11

Topic 4: Choosing Family Wellness Norms...............................13

Topic 5: Aligning Cultural Touch Points....................................18

Topic 6: Mobilizing Peer Support..20

Topic 7: Strengthening the Family Social Climate.....................22

Topic 8: Keeping Relationships Healthy....................................24

Topic 9: Benefiting from Community Resources........................26

Topic 10: Coming Together for Wellness...................................28

Appendix: Copy of Family Member Wellness Portrait Form.......29

Appendix: Copy of Family Wellness Norm Indicator..................30

Appendix: Copy of Cultural Touch Points Indicator...................33

Appendix: Copy of Family Social Climate Indicator..................35

A Family Guide to Wellness: Creating a Family Wellness Culture that Supports Healthy Lifestyles

Copyright © 2011 by Judd Allen

ISBN 978-0-94-1703-32-1

All rights reserved. Printed in the United States of America. No part of this book may be used or reproduced in any manner without written permission except in the case of brief quotations embodied in critical articles and reviews.

Published by

Human Resources Institute, LLC

151 Dunder Road

Burlington, VT 05401 USA

(802) 862-8855

Info@healthyculture.com

www.Healthyculture.com

Quantity purchases of *A Family Guide to Wellness* are available for educational, business and community use.

Photographs available through Istockphoto, LP. The people shown are models used for illustrative purposes only.

Cover photograph of Judd Allen and interior photo of the Allen family by Karen Pike of www.kpikephoto.com. Other cover photographs available through Getty Images. The people shown are models used for illustrative purposes only.

Author Update 2012. *A Family Guide to Wellness* is part of a new initiative called Wellness Culture Coaching.® The initiative is a train-the-trainer system, toolkit and a professional network for those serving as wellness program managers, health coaches and members of wellness committees. Wellness Culture Coaches are empowered to:

(1) Make the case for wellness cultures

(2) Conduct cultural analysis

(3) Develop wellness leaders

(4) Mobilize peer support

(5) Foster household and family wellness cultures

(6) Integrate Wellness Culture Coaching skills and resources into professional practice

The coaching toolkit includes the Lifegain Wellness Culture Survey and report-generating system. It also includes classroom materials and an online training system whereby Wellness Culture Coaches serve as the instructors for wellness leadership, peer support and household/family training.

To learn more or to register for an upcoming Wellness Culture Coach training, visit **wellnessculturecoaching.com.**

« The Family and Wellness Connection »

From birth to death, family has the potential to play a powerful positive role in our well-being.

Our parents and their ancestors are the source of our genetic code. This genetic inheritance contributes greatly to our phsical and psychological disposition.

- Families play important developmental roles throughout our lives. The nurturing we receive as children and the lessons we learn from adults influence our capacity to grow and form healthy relationships with others.

- Families form cultures with their own traditions, expectations and health stories. These cultural influences shape our lifestyles, including whether we are physically active, eat healthy foods and develop close relationships.

Although little can be done about our genetic inheritance, many aspects of family can be organized for wellness. We can, for example, make our family gatherings healthier by including physical activity and healthier food choices. Our family members can also learn to effectively support lifestyle improvement goals. Families can help make wellness a lifelong pursuit; healthy choices can be made for infants, youth, those in middle age, and elders.

« Becoming a Champion of Family Wellness »

This guide introduces tools and strategies for championing wellness in your family. It discusses strategies for mobilizing your family to create a culture that makes healthy lifestyle choices easier to achieve and sustain.

Adopting a culture-based approach to family wellness has a number of unique benefits. When we create a healthy culture, family members benefit just by being part of that culture and, in some instances, living under the same roof. Another great benefit of a family wellness culture is that the natural flow of behavior change is likely to be toward healthier lifestyles. The culture pulls family members in the right direction. This is in stark contrast to the prevailing negative influences in the broader culture, which are leading to growing rates of obesity, inactivity and social isolation. Additionally, a family wellness culture makes positive lifestyle changes stick. You and your family members will achieve greater success with your health improvement goals.

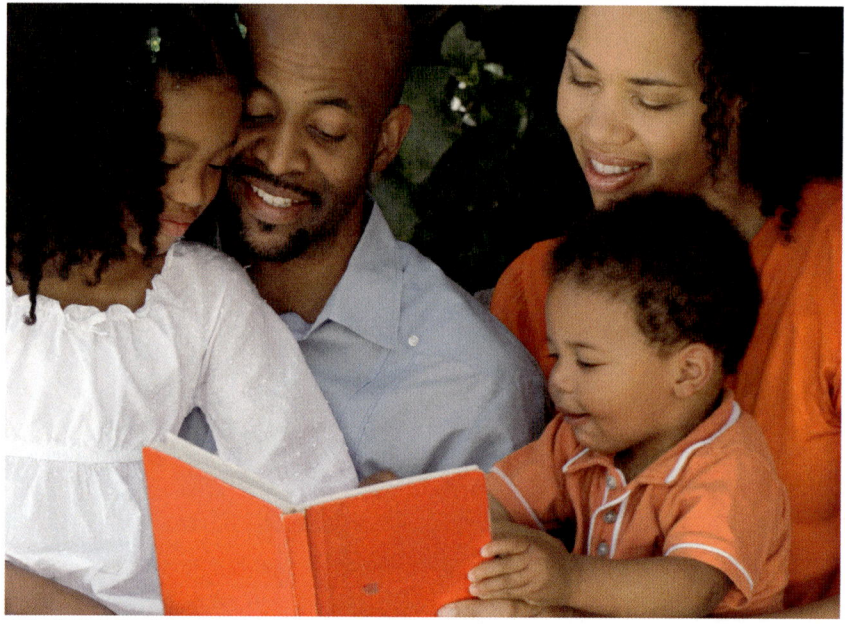

« Topic #1 »
Getting Comfortable with Family Wellness

In American culture, health is commonly viewed as a matter of personal choice. Some people worry about the loss of independence and personal freedom that might result from involving family members in lifestyle goals. These and other objections can be reduced if family members agree to wellness guidelines. Help get everyone on board by discussing the following "starter list" of family wellness guidelines. See if you can agree on those that address the concerns one of more of your family members might have.

- **Family wellness is characterized by mutual support for achieving personal wellness goals.** We want to offer one another encouragement and create the conditions that enable us to achieve our personal wellness goals. We do not need to have the same goals, but we need to find ways to support one another.

- **Family wellness is not psychotherapy or group psychotherapy.** Problems that are deeply rooted or too complex should be handled by health professionals such as counselors or therapists.

- **Family wellness is positive and based on strengths.** We need to build on family history and traditions. We need to learn from and take advantage of the individual skills and knowledge of family members. Ideally, wellness activities should be fun, affirming and meaningful. Successes should be celebrated. Family wellness should not involve pointing fingers and fixing blame.

- **Family wellness mobilizes external support systems.** Workplaces, schools, parks, friends, religious organizations and the community offer valuable wellness programs and activities. We need to find ways to utilize these wellness resources.

« **Topic #2** »

Seeing Your Unique Family System

Families come in all shapes and sizes. You are likely to belong to at least two nuclear families at different times in your life. What kind of family raised you? Perhaps it was a nuclear family. Or maybe you were raised by a single parent with or without the help of extended kin. Maybe you had a stepparent and step- or half-siblings in a blended family. Maybe your family matches none of these descriptions, or it fit different descriptions at different times. It is important to recognize that "family" is experienced in a variety of ways and that each person develops his or her own perceptions of family identity. The mental map of family is constantly evolving as new people enter the family and others depart.

Each person carries an image of his or her family and attitudes toward wellness. Seeing this picture clearly will help you identify key participants in your family wellness initiative. The following questions paint a wellness portrait. Start by answering these questions for each member of your family. Over time you can add to the picture by including information about living and deceased family members you have known. See appendix for a reproducible copy of these questions. Make multiple copies for yourself and other family members.

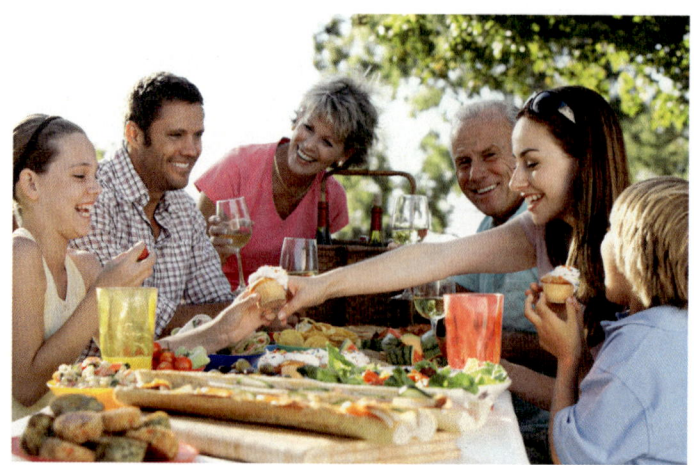

« Family Member Wellness Portrait »

Name of family member _____

Relationship to you _____

On a scale ranging from 10 for very influential to 1 for of little influence, rate the impact this family member has on your life:

10 9 8 7 6 5 4 3 2 1

Thinking broadly about physical, social, economic and emotional dimensions of wellness, how is this family member a good wellness role model? _____
_____

Thinking broadly about physical, social, economic and emotional dimensions of wellness, how is this family member a poor wellness role model? _____
_____

What wellness lessons have you learned as a result of your relationship?
_____
_____

Considering your current wellness goals, how might this family member contribute to your success? _____
_____

How might you assist this family member in achieving his or her wellness goals? _____
_____

« Examining Your Family Wellness Portrait »

One way to use your family portrait is to realize the benefits of wellness role modeling. Hopefully, you have identified a number of ways family members already serve as wellness role models. Keep in mind that a good role model does not have to excel in all aspects of wellness. Sometimes the best role models are people who have overcome wellness challenges and shown that personal change is both possible and worthwhile. We can learn a lot from these wellness stories, particularly if they show how several people pulled together to make a lifestyle change possible. There may be a wellness story in your family that you find informative and inspirational.

It is also likely that the experiences of some of your family members have shown that unhealthy practices can be damaging and sometimes fatal. You may be inspired not to go down the same path. You may be able to see how this family member struggled with unsupportive people and places. It is highly likely that his or her unhealthy behavior could have been remedied with a combination of individual initiative and adequate support. See if you and your family can learn from family illness or tragedy by making sure it is not repeated.

Determine who might play a positive role in supporting and not undermining your current wellness goals. Maybe one of your family members is a particularly good listener or has access to needed resources. Maybe a family member has achieved a similar goal. Maybe someone would be open to joining you in the changes you want to make. You could use a buddy system, checking in regularly and problem solving together.

What if one or more of your family members interfere with your personal wellness? How might you get their support or at least have them agree not to undermine your efforts? For example, if you are pursuing a healthier diet, the cooks in your house need to be on board with your plan. Sometimes it is necessary to reduce exposure to family members who are likely to undermine your wellness.

« Topic #3 »
Developing Your Family's Wellness Story

Creating a family wellness culture is a complex undertaking. Can you create a story of your family living healthfully ever after? Such a plot and storyline could add clarity to your wellness efforts. A wellness story holds the pieces together and helps wellness take root. A meaningful story can add the energy and urgency needed to bring about culture change. A bigger picture of how wellness serves the family elevates the conversation and makes the conversation more about "us" and less about your own personal preferences. Ideally, your family's story will build on what you are already doing, but a wellness story is often a new chapter in the life of the family.

- Sometimes a family's wellness story changes in response to a family crisis such as an illness or death. This might be the case when a heart attack leads to a teachable moment.

- Sometimes a family's wellness story is energized by shared convictions or values. Such would be the case if a family sought to change lifestyle practices to better reflect their shared concerns about the environment.

- Sometimes a family's wellness story turns on the strength of a particularly strong wellness advocate. For example, a mother may become a wellness champion as a result of her concerns about how unhealthy choices will undermine her children's future.

- Sometimes relocation or broader social conditions open up new wellness paths. Many schools, business and communities are taking up wellness causes, addressing, for example, unsafe working conditions, childhood obesity or substance abuse. A family may choose to participate in related wellness activities by becoming more wellness-oriented at home.

« Envisioning Your Family's Wellness Future »

In the space below, summarize your family's wellness story. When it comes to healthy lifestyles and happiness, where have you been and where are you going? How, if at all, do you intend to change the wellness story?

_____

_____

_____

_____

_____

_____

_____

_____

_____

_____

_____

_____

_____

_____

_____

_____

_____

_____

« Topic #4 »

Choosing Family Wellness Norms

Families have their own norms; they are "the way we do things in our family." Family norms are rarely written down and often operate below the radar, coming into view only when someone violates the norm. For example, a family member who decides to stop drinking alcohol or to become a vegetarian might quickly learn that such healthy practices go against how family members are expected to behave. Hopefully, there are some wellness norms firmly in place in your family. For example, a person lighting a cigarette in the house may be asked to smoke outside. On the other hand, some families are so disconnected and geographically spread out that they have few or no cultural norms.

« Family Wellness Norms Indicator »

The following questionnaire assesses important family wellness norms. Your answers will help you identify cultural strengths and opportunities for improvement. This information is needed to set change goals. Using the 5-point scale, rate your level of agreement that the health behavior is the current norm in your immediate family. Keep in mind that we are just asking your opinion and there are no right or wrong answers. Many of these items refer to behaviors that you will view as common sense. This is a positive indication that the particular health behavior is already a strong norm. For some behaviors, there may be no norm. If this is the case, choose 3 for "Neither Agree nor Disagree." Such an answer would indicate that your family culture is not sending strong signals for that healthy lifestyle practice.

See appendix for a reproducible copy of the questionnaire. Make multiple copies for other family members.

« Family Wellness Norms Indicator Continued »

Using the following 5-point scale, rate your level of agreement with the statements below.

5 Strongly Agree
4 Agree
3 Neither Agree nor Disagree
2 Disagree
1 Strongly Disagree

It is normal (expected and accepted) among my immediate family members to...	
Be physically active (such as taking a brisk walk for at least 30 minutes most days).	5 4 3 2 1
Keep flexible through regular stretching.	5 4 3 2 1
Keep muscles in shape through lifting weights or some sort of resistance workout.	5 4 3 2 1
Share fitness equipment.	5 4 3 2 1
Purchase healthy foods.	5 4 3 2 1
Prepare healthy meals.	5 4 3 2 1
Share healthy recipes with each other.	5 4 3 2 1
Maintain a healthy weight by balancing eating and exercise.	5 4 3 2 1
Have a positive attitude.	5 4 3 2 1
Laugh regularly.	5 4 3 2 1
Celebrate personal accomplishments such as the achievement of healthy lifestyle goals.	5 4 3 2 1
Celebrate holidays in healthy ways.	5 4 3 2 1
Vacation in healthy ways.	5 4 3 2 1
Regularly do some healthy activities together.	5 4 3 2 1
Share ideas about things that are both fun and healthy to do.	5 4 3 2 1
Be open to new healthy activities.	5 4 3 2 1
Befriend health-minded peers.	5 4 3 2 1
Join with others in pursuing healthy lifestyle goals.	5 4 3 2 1

« Family Wellness Norms Indicator Continued »

It is normal (expected and accepted) among my immediate family members to…	
Make getting together with friends, family and neighbors a healthy affair.	5 4 3 2 1
Join with others in pursuing healthy lifestyle goals.	5 4 3 2 1
Openly share healthy lifestyle goals.	5 4 3 2 1
Keep the household organized and clean.	5 4 3 2 1
Share household chores.	5 4 3 2 1
Offer assistance to one another.	5 4 3 2 1
Ask for assistance when needed.	5 4 3 2 1
Follow through on commitments.	5 4 3 2 1
Recycle, reuse, turn lights off and otherwise respect the environment.	5 4 3 2 1
Join together for community service or political activities.	5 4 3 2 1
Be financially responsible (such as by paying bills on time and not overspending).	5 4 3 2 1
Get adequate sleep (eight-plus hours) daily.	5 4 3 2 1
Find times to kick back and relax.	5 4 3 2 1
Practice some form of stress management technique (such as yoga, meditation or prayer).	5 4 3 2 1
Take on manageable amounts of responsibility.	5 4 3 2 1
Balance work, rest and play.	5 4 3 2 1
Consume caffeine in a way that does not interfere with rest (such as having less than three cups of coffee daily and well before it is time to sleep).	5 4 3 2 1
Not smoke.	5 4 3 2 1
Avoid smoky places.	5 4 3 2 1
Avoid recreational drug use.	5 4 3 2 1
Never ride in a car that is driven by someone (including myself) who has been drinking or is driving recklessly.	5 4 3 2 1

« Family Wellness Norms Indicator Continued »

It is normal (expected and accepted) among my immediate family members to...	
Drink alcohol moderately, if at all. • For men: consume fewer than 12 drinks per week and fewer than 4 drinks on any single occasion, not exceeding 1 drink per hour. • For women: consume fewer than 9 drinks per week and fewer than 3 drinks on any single occasion, not exceeding 1 drink per hour.	5 4 3 2 1
Wear a seat belt at all times when riding in a car.	5 4 3 2 1
Brush teeth at least twice daily.	5 4 3 2 1
Floss teeth daily.	5 4 3 2 1
Visit a dentist at least once a year.	5 4 3 2 1
Undergo recommended health screenings and physical exams.	5 4 3 2 1
Stay current on vaccinations.	5 4 3 2 1
Respect one another's need for peace and quiet.	5 4 3 2 1
Develop a sense of spirituality, meaning and purpose.	5 4 3 2 1
Respect differences in age, sexual orientation, race, religious beliefs, sex, health, lifestyle, education and political beliefs.	5 4 3 2 1
Have at least one health professional with whom one feels comfortable discussing medical problems.	5 4 3 2 1
Read about health recommendations at the library, in the bookstore or on the Internet.	5 4 3 2 1
Be a careful consumer of medical resources by getting second opinions where appropriate, following through on treatment plans and asking about costs.	5 4 3 2 1
Rest and take time to recover when sick.	5 4 3 2 1

« Scoring the Family Wellness Norms Indicator »

Step 1: Identify Wellness Strengths

Determine which norms received a score of 4 or 5. These are your family culture's wellness strengths. It will be relatively easy for a given member of your family to achieve personal goals that are consistent with these strong positive norms.

We can learn a lot from our strengths. Think about how these norms became firmly established in your family. Perhaps you can repeat this technique to strengthen norms that need changing.

Step 2: Identify Unhealthy Norms

Identify behaviors for which the norms do not support healthy practices. Typically, these are the behaviors you rated as 3 or less on the 5-point scale.

Step 3: Select Norm Goals

Changing norms requires considerable focus and follow-through. Ideally, you and your family members will agree on one or two priorities for new wellness norms. Additional goals can be set in the coming months. Your initial family wellness norm goals will help you address shared health concerns and establish your family's wellness culture. For example, you may determine that it should be a norm to cut television time to an hour or less daily. Another example would be to establish a new norm for incorporating physical activity into family holiday activities and vacations. Such norms would define your family's wellness culture.

« Topic #5 »
Aligning Cultural Touch Points

Family norms are established and reinforced through a variety of social mechanisms called cultural touch points. Few, if any, of these social influences are written down. They include such things as rewards, recognition, traditions, and the commitment of family resources.

« Cultural Touch Points Indicator »

The following Cultural Touch Points Indicator helps clarify how touch points support wellness in your family. By understanding and using touch points, you and your family will be better positioned to achieve the norm goals you identified in the previous exercise. See appendix for a reproducible copy of the questions. Make multiple copies for other family members.

Using the 5-point scale, rate your level of agreement with the following statements.

5 Strongly Agree
4 Agree
3 Neither Agree nor Disagree
2 Disagree
1 Strongly Disagree

My family demonstrates its commitment to supporting healthy lifestyles through its use of resources such as time, space and money.	5 4 3 2 1
We set aside money for healthy activities (such as up-to-date fitness equipment, health club memberships and subscriptions to health information resources).	5 4 3 2 1
Family members are rewarded and recognized for efforts to live a healthy lifestyle.	5 4 3 2 1

Unhealthy behaviors such as physical inactivity, overeating, smoking and excess drinking are discouraged.	5 4 3 2 1
Healthy behaviors such as stress management, exercise and healthy eating are almost never discouraged.	5 4 3 2 1
My family models healthy lifestyles.	5 4 3 2 1
We teach each other skills needed to achieve a healthy lifestyle.	5 4 3 2 1
New members of our family are made aware of our interest in healthy lifestyles.	5 4 3 2 1
Our social times tend to include activities such as healthy eating or exercise.	5 4 3 2 1
We have one or more traditions or rituals that symbolize our commitment to healthy lifestyles.	5 4 3 2 1
Family members have access to health assessments and medical screenings that provide feedback on how they are doing in terms of living a healthy lifestyle.	5 4 3 2 1

Questions for Family Members Living Together

We have organized our household's physical environment to support wellness by, for example, setting aside space for exercise equipment and quiet areas for relaxation.	5 4 3 2 1
Our home is stocked with healthy foods.	5 4 3 2 1

« Interpreting the Cultural Touch Points Indicator »

Your responses to the Cultural Touch Points Indicator quantify the strength of your family wellness culture. Most families do not achieve a perfect score of 5 on all questions. Your goal is to get most of these cultural influences working for wellness. Now that you have an overall picture, you can determine how touch points can be better aligned with wellness. Your plan for creating a wellness culture will include recommendations for strengthening positive cultural influences and for weakening negative cultural influences.

« Topic #6 »
Mobilizing Peer Support

Each year, most people attempt to achieve at least one lifestyle improvement goal. The most common goals are losing weight, eating a healthier diet, getting physically fit and managing stress. Unfortunately, few of these goals are achieved, often because we lack the support we need to follow through on them. Family members can be an important source of support. At the very least, they can help by not standing in the way.

The first step to increasing the quality and quantity of support in your family is to develop a regular time and place for ongoing conversations about lifestyle improvement. For example, you could make it a tradition to talk about healthy lifestyle goals during the evening meal. Most days this conversation could be a simple check-in, and one mealtime each week could be designated for a longer conversation. The following topics are good subjects for the longer conversations.

Topics for Family Conversations about Peer Support

- When two or more family members have similar lifestyle goals, a buddy system increases opportunities for mutual support. What will be done to establish a wellness buddy system in our family?

- A family member may benefit from conversations with someone who has achieved similar lifestyle goals under similar circumstances. How will we support housemates in their efforts to find good role models?

- Many lifestyle changes require resources such as time, space, mental focus and equipment. How will we help our family members get the resources they need and eliminate barriers to lifestyle improvement?

- Physical and social environments can either undermine or support healthy lifestyles. How will we help our family members find or create supportive environments for their desired practices?

- It is common to falter in making a lifestyle change. How will we help our family members reduce and manage high-risk situations so that they can avoid relapse into unhealthy practices? How will we help our family members get back on track when they have a setback?

- Too many successes go unacknowledged. How will we recognize and celebrate the progress we make in achieving our goals?

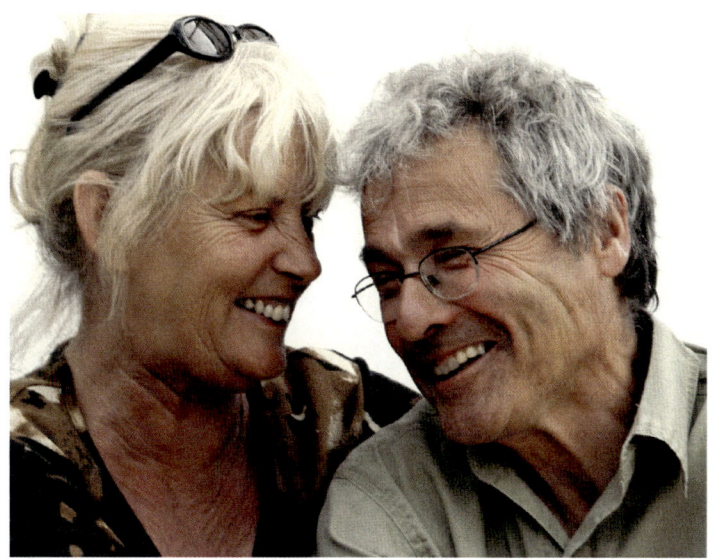

« Topic #7 »
Strengthening the Family Social Climate

It is hard to be well in a hostile family environment. This is obvious to a family going through an acrimonious divorce. It is equally true when family members have become distant and disconnected. Wellness goals get pushed to the side.

Creating a healthy and productive family social climate is an important goal of family wellness. Such climates tend to have a strong sense of community, a shared vision and a positive outlook. The following Family Social Climate Indicator will help you assess the social atmosphere in your family.

See appendix for a reproducible copy of the questions. Make multiple copies for other family members.

« Family Social Climate Indicator »

Using the 5-point scale, rate your level of agreement with the following statements.

> 5 Strongly Agree
> 4 Agree
> 3 Neither Agree nor Disagree
> 2 Disagree
> 1 Strongly Disagree

We care for one another in times of need.	5 4 3 2 1
We stay current on one another's activities and interests.	5 4 3 2 1
We have really gotten to know one another.	5 4 3 2 1
We trust one another.	5 4 3 2 1
We feel comfortable saying what is on our minds.	5 4 3 2 1

« Family Social Climate Indicator Continued »

We look forward to a future together.	5 4 3 2 1
We feel a strong sense of belonging.	5 4 3 2 1
We share common values.	5 4 3 2 1
We listen to one another.	5 4 3 2 1
We make decisions in inclusive and respectful ways.	5 4 3 2 1
We cooperate with one another.	5 4 3 2 1
We share responsibility for making the family work.	5 4 3 2 1
We have clear and consistent family goals.	5 4 3 2 1
We give one another the freedom to do things in our own way.	5 4 3 2 1
We have a high level of team spirit.	5 4 3 2 1
We resolve conflict in positive ways.	5 4 3 2 1
We celebrate achievements.	5 4 3 2 1
We have a "can do" attitude.	5 4 3 2 1
We are proud of our family.	5 4 3 2 1

« Interpreting the Family Social Climate Indicator »

Few families achieve a score of 5 on all items. You and your family members can use the answers to identify ways to improve the climate. If most individual item scores are 3 or lower, your family social climate is probably undermining wellness. If you have such low scores, improving the climate should be the immediate priority; an improved climate will be needed to achieve wellness goals.

« Topic #8 »
Keeping Relationships Healthy

Healthy relationships are the building blocks of a supportive culture. Healthy relationships are based on kindness, mutual understanding and trust. They allow people the freedom to grow and to enjoy each other's company.

Unfortunately, past experiences in dysfunctional social groups and relationships make many of us slow to embrace the power and benefits of achieving wellness together. Bad social experiences can lead us to resist social ties. The fear is that we will become dependent on others and that this will undermine our personal responsibility and freedom. The best way to allay this fear is to keep track of the relationships you have with your family to make sure they are still healthy.

- **Are family members doing more talking than listening?** Helpful relationships primarily involve asking useful questions and listening, not being a "know-it-all." Look at the balance of questions and advice. If a family member is growing tired of getting advice, then the relationship may be tipping into disempowerment mode. Change the mix.

- **Do any family members feel overcommitted?** Helping others should not feel like a burden. Having too many responsibilities can lead to a lack of follow-through. If people are overcommitted, they are probably giving less than their full attention to their family members. Family members should be able to maintain their wellness and personal priorities.

- **Is there equality?** In American culture, there is a tendency to look down on people who need help. It is difficult, given this tradition, to view those being helped as equals. It can be difficult to refrain from seeing the giving of help as a rationale for having power over a family member.

- **Is dependency developing?** There is a line beyond which helping someone undermines his or her capabilities. Family members need to come up with their own solutions to their problems; they should not be spoon-fed solutions. Family members should make decisions and develop a sense of responsibility. If the line has been crossed and the person being helped has developed feelings of dependency, it is time to reassess.

- **Is someone obsessed with goals**? Wellness goals are important, but sometimes it is okay to move on to other issues or delay change for a little while. If family members are becoming angry, frustrated or annoyed about lack of progress, it may be time to reassess.

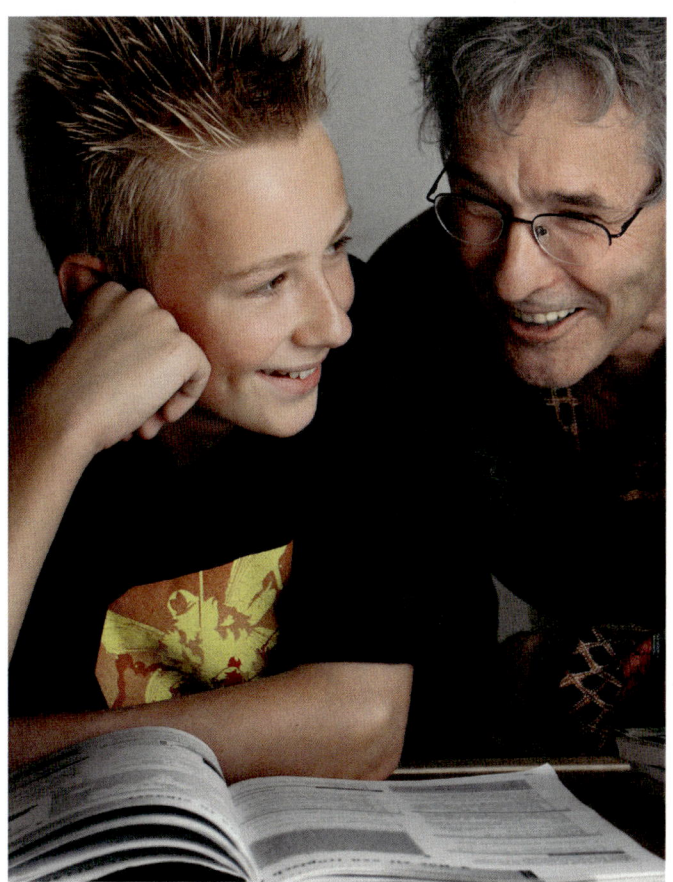

« Topic #9 »

Benefiting from Community Resources

Families can tap into community wellness resources. The obesity epidemic, an aging population, and skyrocketing health-care costs are driving a lot of interest in healthy lifestyles. The majority of employers and insurance companies now offer wellness programs. These programs often include personal health assessments, health coaching, informative websites, and educational programs. Schools are taking a new look at the need for healthy eating and physical activity. Some schools have eliminated or reduced vending machines that sell high-calorie and salty products. Community organizations, such as the YMCA, yoga studios and health clubs, are also contributing to wellness conversations and resources. Grocery stores have begun improving their product labeling by offering easier-to-understand health scores. The following checklist will help you locate wellness resources that could benefit your family.

« Community Resource Checklist »

- If one or more of your family members work outside the home, find out what worksite wellness programs are available and determine the rules regarding family use of these resources. Many employers offer such valuable resources as discounts to fitness facilities. See how your family can get in on these important benefits.

- If one or more of your family members have health insurance, find out what wellness programs are being offered through the insurer. Many insurance companies are ramping up their wellness offerings; company representatives can explain them to you or send you to a website listing these resources.

- Health-care organizations such as hospitals frequently offer educational programs related to wellness. To find out more, call the health-care organization and ask to speak with the people responsible for health promotion and wellness.

- YMCAs and other health clubs frequently offer wellness services. Although the primary emphasis is on physical activity, many such clubs offer programs for stress management and weight controlIf you or another family member would benefit from professional support, these organizations are a good place to start. They often have listings and/or contracts with nutritionists, wellness coaches and personal trainers.

- Most communities have wellness support groups such as Alcoholics Anonymous, Weight Watchers and Jenny Craig. You can search for these local resources on the Internet or in the phone book.

- Schools may have wellness education programs that are available to students' family members. Some colleges and universities make health-related lectures available to community members. They may offer courses on such topics as healthy cooking, triathlon training and positive psychology.

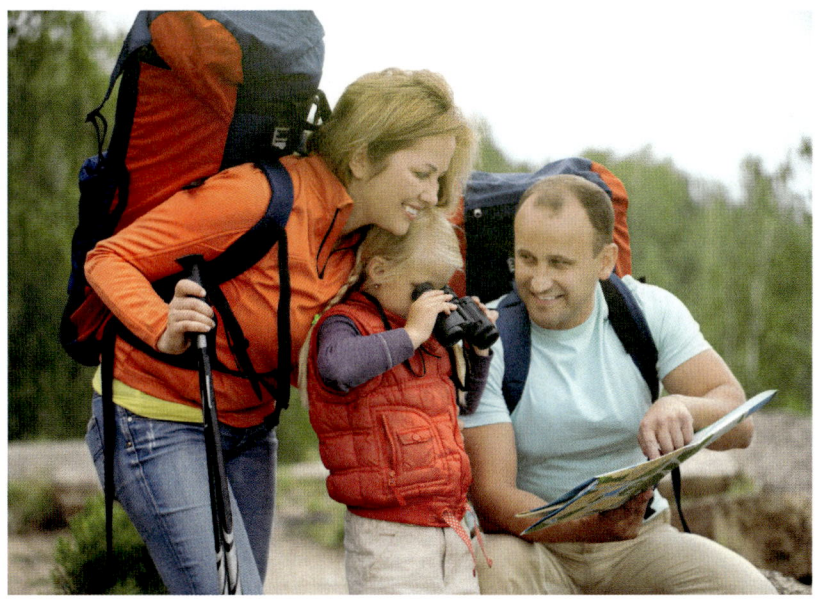

« Topic #10 »

Coming Together for Wellness

There is perhaps no finer gift or greater purpose than helping those you love achieve a long, happy and healthy life. A wellness focus adds value to our family relationships. When we help one another achieve wellness goals, we are showing kindness and expressing love. When we join together to create conditions that make the healthy choice the easier choice, we are proving that our families can achieve more together than any one family member could achieve on his or her own. This is further evidence that our biological need for each other is not an obstacle to overcome, but rather a virtue to be celebrated.

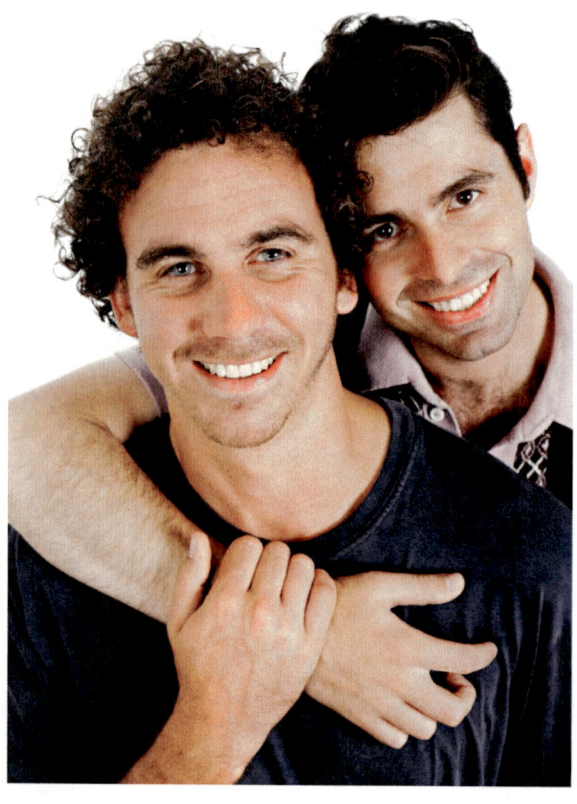

Appendix
« Family Member Wellness Portrait »

Name of family member _____

Relationship to you _____

On a scale ranging from 10 for very influential to 1 for of little influence, rate the impact this family member has on your life:

10 9 8 7 6 5 4 3 2 1

Thinking broadly about physical, social, economic and emotional dimensions of wellness, how is this family member a good wellness role model? _____
_____

Thinking broadly about physical, social, economic and emotional dimensions of wellness, how is this family member a poor wellness role model? _____
_____

What wellness lessons have you learned as a result of your relationship?
_____
_____

Considering your current wellness goals, how might this family member contribute to your success? _____
_____

How might you assist this family member in achieving his or her wellness goals? _____
_____

Reproduce this page to complete portraits for each family member.

Appendix
« Family Wellness Norm Indicator »

Using the 5-point scale, rate your level of agreement with the following statements.

>   5 Strongly Agree
>   4 Agree
>   3 Neither Agree nor Disagree
>   2 Disagree
>   1 Strongly Disagree

It is normal (expected and accepted) among my immediate family members to...	
Be physically active (such as taking a brisk walk for at least 30 minutes most days).	5 4 3 2 1
Keep flexible through regular stretching.	5 4 3 2 1
Keep muscles in shape through lifting weights or some sort of resistance workout.	5 4 3 2 1
Share fitness equipment.	5 4 3 2 1
Purchase healthy foods.	5 4 3 2 1
Prepare healthy meals.	5 4 3 2 1
Share healthy recipes with each other.	5 4 3 2 1
Maintain a healthy weight by balancing eating and exercise.	5 4 3 2 1
Have a positive attitude.	5 4 3 2 1
Laugh regularly.	5 4 3 2 1
Celebrate personal accomplishments such as the achievement of healthy lifestyle goals.	5 4 3 2 1
Celebrate holidays in healthy ways.	5 4 3 2 1
Vacation in healthy ways.	5 4 3 2 1
Regularly do some healthy activities together.	5 4 3 2 1
Share ideas about things that are both fun and healthy to do.	5 4 3 2 1
Be open to new healthy activities.	5 4 3 2 1
Befriend health-minded peers.	5 4 3 2 1

« Family Wellness Norm Indicator Continued »

It is normal (expected and accepted) among my immediate family members to...	
Make getting together with friends, family and neighbors a healthy affair.	5 4 3 2 1
Join with others in pursuing healthy lifestyle goals.	5 4 3 2 1
Openly share healthy lifestyle goals.	5 4 3 2 1
Keep the household organized and clean.	5 4 3 2 1
Share household chores.	5 4 3 2 1
Offer assistance to one another.	5 4 3 2 1
Ask for assistance when needed.	5 4 3 2 1
Follow through on commitments.	5 4 3 2 1
Recycle, reuse, turn lights off and otherwise respect the environment.	5 4 3 2 1
Join together for community service or political activities.	5 4 3 2 1
Be financially responsible (such as by paying bills on time and not overspending).	5 4 3 2 1
Get adequate sleep (eight-plus hours) daily.	5 4 3 2 1
Find times to kick back and relax.	5 4 3 2 1
Practice some form of stress management technique (such as yoga, meditation or prayer).	5 4 3 2 1
Take on manageable amounts of responsibility.	5 4 3 2 1
Balance work, rest and play.	5 4 3 2 1
Consume caffeine in a way that does not interfere with rest (such as having less than three cups of coffee daily and well before it is time to sleep).	5 4 3 2 1
Not smoke.	5 4 3 2 1
Avoid smoky places.	5 4 3 2 1
Avoid recreational drug use.	5 4 3 2 1
Never ride in a car that is driven by someone (including myself) who has been drinking or is driving recklessly.	5 4 3 2 1

« Family Wellness Norm Indicator Continued »

It is normal (expected and accepted) among my immediate family members to...	
Drink alcohol moderately, if at all. • For men: consume fewer than 12 drinks per week and fewer than 4 drinks on any single occasion, not exceeding 1 drink per hour. • For women: consume fewer than 9 drinks per week and fewer than 3 drinks on any single occasion, not exceeding 1 drink per hour.	5 4 3 2 1
Wear a seat belt at all times when riding in a car.	5 4 3 2 1
Brush teeth at least twice daily.	5 4 3 2 1
Floss teeth daily.	5 4 3 2 1
Visit a dentist at least once a year.	5 4 3 2 1
Undergo recommended health screenings and physical exams.	5 4 3 2 1
Stay current on vaccinations.	5 4 3 2 1
Respect one another's need for peace and quiet.	5 4 3 2 1
Develop a sense of spirituality, meaning and purpose.	5 4 3 2 1
Respect differences in age, sexual orientation, race, religious beliefs, sex, health, lifestyle, education and political beliefs.	5 4 3 2 1
Have at least one health professional with whom one feels comfortable discussing medical problems.	5 4 3 2 1
Read about health recommendations at the library, in the bookstore or on the Internet.	5 4 3 2 1
Be a careful consumer of medical resources by getting second opinions where appropriate, following through on treatment plans and asking about costs.	5 4 3 2 1
Rest and take time to recover when sick.	5 4 3 2 1

Appendix
« Cultural Touch Points Indicator »

The following Cultural Touch Points Indicator helps clarify how touch points support wellness in your family. Using the 5-point scale, rate your level of agreement with the following statements.

        5 Strongly Agree
        4 Agree
        3 Neither Agree nor Disagree
        2 Disagree
        1 Strongly Disagree

My family demonstrates its commitment to supporting healthy lifestyles through its use of resources such as time, space and money.	5 4 3 2 1
We set aside money for healthy activities (such as up-to-date fitness equipment, health club memberships and subscriptions to health information resources).	5 4 3 2 1
Family members are rewarded and recognized for efforts to live a healthy lifestyle.	5 4 3 2 1
Unhealthy behaviors such as physical inactivity, overeating, smoking and excess drinking are discouraged.	5 4 3 2 1
Healthy behaviors such as stress management, exercise and healthy eating are almost never discouraged.	5 4 3 2 1
My family models healthy lifestyles.	5 4 3 2 1
We teach each other skills needed to achieve a healthy lifestyle.	5 4 3 2 1
New members of our family are made aware of our interest in healthy lifestyles.	5 4 3 2 1
Our social times tend to include activities such as healthy eating or exercise.	5 4 3 2 1
We have one or more traditions or rituals that symbolize our commitment to healthy lifestyles.	5 4 3 2 1
Family members have access to health assessments and medical screenings that provide feedback on how they are doing in terms of living a healthy lifestyle	5 4 3 2 1

« Cultural Touch Points Indicator Continued »

Questions for Family Members Living Together

We have organized our household's physical environment to support wellness by, for example, setting aside space for exercise equipment and quiet areas for relaxation.	5 4 3 2 1
Our home is stocked with healthy foods.	5 4 3 2 1

Appendix
« Family Social Climate Indicator »

Using the 5-point scale, rate your level of agreement with the following statements.

> 5 Strongly Agree
> 4 Agree
> 3 Neither Agree nor Disagree
> 2 Disagree
> 1 Strongly Disagree

We care for one another in times of need.	5 4 3 2 1
We stay current on one another's activities and interests.	5 4 3 2 1
We have really gotten to know one another.	5 4 3 2 1
We trust one another.	5 4 3 2 1
We feel comfortable saying what is on our minds.	5 4 3 2 1
We look forward to a future together.	5 4 3 2 1
We feel a strong sense of belonging.	5 4 3 2 1
We share common values.	5 4 3 2 1
We listen to one another.	5 4 3 2 1
We make decisions in inclusive and respectful ways.	5 4 3 2 1
We cooperate with one another.	5 4 3 2 1
We share responsibility for making the family work.	5 4 3 2 1
We have clear and consistent family goals.	5 4 3 2 1
We give one another the freedom to do things in our own way.	5 4 3 2 1
We have a high level of team spirit.	5 4 3 2 1
We resolve conflict in positive ways.	5 4 3 2 1
We celebrate achievements.	5 4 3 2 1
We have a "can do" attitude.	5 4 3 2 1
We are proud of our family.	5 4 3 2 1

Also by Judd Allen, Ph.D.

Bringing Wellness Home is for anyone living with others. Bringing Wellness Home guides efforts to: (1) choose the household wellness norms you want and need, (2) create a shared vision for wellness at home, (3) align cultural influences such as traditions and rewards, (4) develop peer support skills that nurture positive and lasting lifestyle change, (5) foster a caring and fun household climate.

Kitchen Table Talks for Wellness features 15 great conversations about creating a household culture that supports healthy lifestyles. Each chapter reviews key ideas such establishing wellness traditions and then offers questions that address the wellness strategy.

Healthy Habits, Helpful Friends empowers peers to assist with lifestyle change. In addition to learning how to lay a solid foundation for effective peer support, readers learn skills for: (1) setting wellness goals, (2) locating ideal role models, (3) eliminating barriers to change, (4) finding or creating supportive environments, (5) avoiding relapse, and (6) celebrating success.

Wellness Leadership empowers managers, wellness committee members and other wellness champions to create a workplace culture that supports healthy lifestyles. Such a culture of health saves lives, cuts medical costs, enhances productivity, improves morale and adds new vitality to work groups. *Wellness Leadership* explains how to create a shared wellness vision, serve as an effective role model, align cultural influences and monitor/celebrate success. Revealing self-tests, a culture survey, information about legal issues, guidelines for establishing wellness committees, leadership stories and checklists take the guesswork out of creating a culture of health.

The books can be ordered using the following form or at www.healthyculture.com. Call (802) 862-8855 for information about volume discounts.

Quick Book Order Form

$14.95 each. Any two books for $24.95. Call for quantity pricing. US Shipping: $3.95 for first book. Fee shipping on additional US orders. $9 charge for the first two books shipped outside the US.

Please add 8% sales tax for books shipped to a Vermont address.

Please indicate the number of books below:

    ____ Wellness Leadership

    ____ Bringing Wellness Home

    ____ Healthy Habits, Helpful Friends

    ____ Kitchen Table Talks for Wellness

    ____ A Family Guide to Wellness

Name

Address

Billing address if other than shipping address

Telephone

Email

We gladly accept checks in U.S. funds payable to the Human Resources Institute, LLC

MasterCard or VISA Card Number _____

Expiration date _____

Fax orders: 802-862-6389

Telephone orders: 802-862-8855

Email orders: Info@healthyculture.com

Send postal orders to Healthyculture.com, 151 Dunder Road, Burlington, Vermont, 05401 USA

Made in United States
Orlando, FL
19 June 2024